XKHORT COMEDY

EMBRACING BLISS

Discovering the 5 Secrets to a GOODLIFE"

Contents

WHAT IS LIFE

Life is a complex phenomenon characterized by the ability to grow, reproduce, and adapt to the environment. It involves living organisms that exhibit various biological processes such as metabolism, response to stimuli, and the capacity for evolution.

WHAT IS GOOD-LIFE

Good life typically refers to a state of well-being, contentment, and fulfillment. It can vary from person to person, but generally, it involves a balance between physical health, emotional well-being, meaningful relationships, personal growth, and a sense of purpose or satisfaction in life. It is subjective and can be influenced by cultural, societal, and individual values and beliefs.

Certainly! A good life is a concept that has been explored and discussed by philosophers, psychologists, and thinkers throughout history. It involves several key aspects:

1. Physical Health: A good life often includes having good physical health, which allows you to enjoy daily activities, pursue interests, and have the energy to engage with the world.

2. Emotional Well-being: Emotional well-being involves having a positive and stable emotional state, experiencing happiness, joy, and managing negative emotions effectively.
3. Meaningful Relationships: Having meaningful and supportive relationships with family, friends, and a broader community is crucial for a good life. These connections provide social support, love, and a sense of belonging.
4. Personal Growth: Continuous learning, self-improvement, and the pursuit of personal goals and aspirations contribute to a fulfilling life.
5. Purpose and Satisfaction: Feeling a sense of purpose, meaning, and accomplishment in one's actions and contributions can lead to a greater sense of fulfillment.
6. Work-Life Balance: Finding a balance between work, leisure, and personal life is essential to avoid burnout and maintain overall well-being.
7. Values and Beliefs: Aligning actions with personal values and beliefs can bring a sense of integrity and authenticity to life.

It's important to note that the definition of a good life is subjective and can vary based on individual experiences, cultural backgrounds, and personal preferences. Ultimately, it is about finding a balance and living a life that brings happiness and satisfaction while being mindful of the needs of others and the impact on the world around us.

Three

SECRET OF GOOD-LIFE

1. Gratitude
2. Mindfulness
3. Giving Back
4. Pursuit of Passions
5. Embracing Change

THE FIRST SECRET

GRATITUDE is the practice of being thankful and appreciative for the positive aspects of life, both big and small. It involves recognizing and acknowledging the good things that happen, the kindness of others, and the positive experiences that come our way.

Practicing gratitude can have several positive effects on a person's well-being:

1. Positive Outlook: Gratitude helps shift the focus from negative thoughts to positive ones, fostering a more optimistic outlook on life.
2. Emotional Resilience: It can increase emotional resilience, making it easier to cope with challenges and setbacks.
3. Improved Relationships: Expressing gratitude towards others strengthens relationships, as it shows appreciation and enhances feelings of connection.

4. Stress Reduction: Being grateful can reduce stress and anxiety levels by promoting a sense of calm and contentment.
5. Better Sleep: Cultivating gratitude before bedtime has been linked to improved sleep quality.

Ways to practice gratitude include keeping a gratitude journal, regularly expressing thanks to others, reflecting on positive experiences, or simply taking a moment each day to appreciate the things we often take for granted.

Incorporating gratitude into daily life can significantly contribute to an individual's overall happiness and well-being, making it an essential element of a good life.

Certainly! Here are some additional insights and benefits about the practice of gratitude:

1. Enhanced Mental Health: Gratitude has been associated with a reduction in symptoms of depression and anxiety. By focusing on positive aspects, it can counteract negative thought patterns.
2. Physical Health Benefits: Practicing gratitude may lead to improved physical health. Studies have shown that grateful individuals tend to engage in healthier behaviors such as regular exercise and better nutrition.
3. Strengthened Relationships: Expressing gratitude and appreciation can deepen connections with others. It fosters a positive atmosphere and reinforces feelings of trust and mutual respect.
4. Increased Resilience: Grateful individuals often exhibit greater resilience during challenging times. They are more likely to find strength and learn valuable lessons from

difficult experiences.

5. Dopamine Boost: Expressing gratitude triggers the release of dopamine, the "feel-good" neurotransmitter, which reinforces the positive behavior of being thankful.

6. Gratitude's Ripple Effect: Gratitude has a ripple effect, where expressing thanks can inspire others to do the same, creating a more positive and uplifting environment.

7. Stress Reduction: By focusing on what we are grateful for, we divert attention from worries and stressors, leading to reduced stress and an increased sense of calm.

8. Increased Satisfaction: Gratitude helps individuals focus on what they have, rather than what they lack, leading to greater satisfaction with life.

9. Strengthened Emotional Bonds: Gratitude can strengthen emotional bonds between family members, friends, and colleagues, contributing to a more supportive and harmonious social environment.

10. Mindfulness and Gratitude: Practicing mindfulness and gratitude together can create a powerful synergy. Being present in the moment helps individuals appreciate and savor the positive experiences in their lives.

Overall, gratitude is a simple yet powerful practice that has the potential to transform one's perspective, enrich relationships, and contribute to a fulfilling and meaningful life. Embracing gratitude as a daily habit can have a profound and positive impact on both mental and physical well-being.

Five

THE SECOND SECRET

"MINDFULNESS" refers to the practice of being fully present and aware of the current moment without judgment. It involves paying attention to your thoughts, feelings, bodily sensations, and the environment around you with an attitude of openness and curiosity.

Key aspects of mindfulness:

1. Present-Moment Awareness: Mindfulness encourages focusing on the present moment without dwelling on the past or worrying about the future. It helps individuals become more attuned to their experiences as they unfold.

2. Non-Judgmental Attitude: Mindfulness involves accepting thoughts and feelings without labeling them as good or bad. It's about observing experiences objectively, without criticizing oneself for having certain thoughts or emotions.

3. Increased Self-Awareness: Through mindfulness, individ-

uals gain a deeper understanding of their thought patterns, emotions, and reactions. This self-awareness can lead to better emotional regulation and decision-making.

4. Stress Reduction: Mindfulness practices, such as meditation, have been shown to reduce stress and anxiety. By focusing on the present and letting go of worries, individuals can experience a sense of calm and relaxation.

5. Improved Concentration: Mindfulness exercises can enhance concentration and focus by training the mind to stay attentive to the task at hand.

6. Enhanced Emotional Resilience: Mindfulness helps individuals respond to challenges with greater emotional resilience, as they learn to acknowledge and accept difficult emotions without becoming overwhelmed by them.

7. Better Interpersonal Relationships: Mindful listening and communication can improve relationships by promoting empathy and understanding.

8. Positive Mental Health: Regular mindfulness practices have been linked to improved overall mental well-being and a decreased risk of depression and other mental health issues.

Practicing mindfulness can take many forms, such as mindfulness meditation, deep breathing exercises, body scanning, and mindful movement like yoga. By incorporating mindfulness into daily life, individuals can cultivate a greater sense of inner peace, reduce stress, and foster a more positive and balanced outlook on life.

Certainly! Here are some additional insights and benefits related to the practice of mindfulness:

1. Increased Emotional Regulation: Mindfulness helps individuals become more aware of their emotions as they arise. By observing emotions without judgment, people can develop better emotional regulation skills, leading to healthier responses to challenging situations.
2. Reduced Rumination: Mindfulness can break the cycle of repetitive and negative thinking, reducing rumination and promoting a clearer and more focused mind.
3. Greater Compassion: Mindfulness practices often cultivate a sense of compassion, both for oneself and others. This increased empathy can lead to more caring and supportive relationships.
4. Mindful Eating: Applying mindfulness to eating habits can lead to healthier food choices, improved digestion, and a better understanding of hunger and fullness cues.
5. Improved Sleep: Practicing mindfulness before bedtime can relax the mind and body, leading to improved sleep quality and better rest.
6. Pain Management: Mindfulness-based interventions have been found effective in managing chronic pain conditions by changing individuals' perception of pain and reducing its impact on daily life.
7. Cognitive Flexibility: Mindfulness can enhance cognitive flexibility, allowing individuals to adapt and problem-solve more effectively.
8. Mindful Parenting: Mindfulness practices can benefit parents by helping them be more present and attentive to their children, leading to stronger parent-child relationships.
9. Workplace Benefits: Incorporating mindfulness in the workplace has been shown to reduce stress, enhance focus, and improve overall job satisfaction and productivity.

10. Mindfulness for Anxiety: Mindfulness-based therapies have proven helpful for managing anxiety disorders, providing individuals with tools to navigate anxious thoughts and feelings.
11. Improved Memory: Regular mindfulness practice has been linked to improved memory and cognitive functioning.
12. Self-Compassion: Mindfulness encourages individuals to treat themselves with kindness and understanding, fostering a sense of self-compassion and self-acceptance.

Remember, mindfulness is a skill that requires practice and patience. It is not about eliminating all thoughts or emotions but about observing them with curiosity and non-judgment. Integrating mindfulness into daily life can lead to numerous physical, mental, and emotional benefits, ultimately contributing to a more fulfilling and balanced life.

Six

THE THIRD SECRET

"GIVING BACK," involves engaging in acts of kindness, generosity, and making positive contributions to others and the community. It is the practice of sharing resources, time, or skills with the intention of benefiting others without expecting anything in return.

Key aspects of giving back:

1. Acts of Kindness: Giving back can include small acts of kindness like helping a neighbor, offering a listening ear to a friend, or expressing gratitude to someone who made a difference in your life.
2. Volunteering: Volunteering your time and skills to support charitable organizations, community initiatives, or causes can have a significant impact on those in need.
3. Philanthropy: Donating money or resources to support various charitable causes and organizations can make a

positive difference in people's lives.

4. Paying It Forward: The concept of paying it forward involves doing something kind for others with the hope that they, in turn, will do something kind for someone else.

5. Environmental Impact: Giving back can also extend to caring for the environment, such as participating in clean-up initiatives or adopting sustainable practices to reduce ecological footprints.

Benefits of giving back:

1. Sense of Purpose: Contributing to the well-being of others and the community can provide a sense of purpose and meaning in life.

2. Increased Happiness: Studies have shown that acts of kindness and giving back can lead to increased levels of happiness and well-being.

3. Strengthened Empathy: Engaging in acts of giving can enhance empathy and understanding towards others' experiences and struggles.

4. Building Community: Giving back fosters a sense of community and social connectedness as individuals come together to support common causes.

5. Positive Impact: By giving back, individuals have the opportunity to make a positive impact on the lives of others, no matter how big or small.

6. Personal Growth: Engaging in giving back activities can lead to personal growth and a broader perspective on life, as it exposes individuals to different perspectives and challenges.

7. Enhanced Gratitude: Giving back can deepen feelings of gratitude for one's own circumstances and privileges.
8. Ripple Effect: Acts of kindness and giving can create a ripple effect, inspiring others to do the same, creating a more compassionate and caring society.

Giving back not only benefits the recipients but also positively affects the giver, leading to a more fulfilling and interconnected life. Whether through small gestures of kindness or larger charitable contributions, the act of giving back has the power to create positive change in the world and leave a lasting impact on individuals and communities alike.

Certainly! Giving back, also known as altruism or philanthropy, is a timeless and universal practice that transcends cultures and societies. It embodies the spirit of selflessness, compassion, and a desire to improve the lives of others and contribute to the greater good. While the act of giving back has numerous benefits for both the recipients and the giver, it goes beyond just material or financial contributions. Let's delve deeper into the significance and impact of giving back in various aspects of life.

1. Sense of Purpose and Meaning: Giving back can offer a profound sense of purpose and meaning in life. Knowing that one's actions positively influence the lives of others can provide a deep and fulfilling sense of satisfaction, leading to a greater sense of purpose.
2. Enhanced Well-Being and Happiness: Studies have consistently shown that engaging in acts of kindness and altruism can lead to increased levels of happiness and overall well-being. The act of giving activates areas of

the brain associated with pleasure and reward, creating a sense of joy and fulfillment.

3. Strengthened Empathy and Compassion: Regularly giving back can cultivate and strengthen empathy and compassion towards others. By understanding and responding to the needs of those less fortunate, individuals develop a deeper connection to the human experience and a greater appreciation for the struggles and challenges others face.

4. Building Community and Social Bonds: Giving back fosters a sense of community and social disconnectedness. Whether participating in local community projects, supporting charitable organizations, or collaborating with others for a common cause, the act of giving brings people together to address shared concerns and work towards a collective goal.

5. Positive Impact on Mental Health: Engaging in acts of altruism has been associated with reduced levels of stress, anxiety, and depression. The act of giving triggers the release of neurotransmitters like Oxycontin and endorphins, which promote feelings of happiness, trust, and bonding.

6. Personal Growth and Development: Giving back offers opportunities for personal growth and self-improvement. It encourages individuals to step outside their comfort zones, develop new skills, and broaden their perspectives by interacting with diverse groups of people and understanding different social issues.

7. Inspiring Others: Acts of kindness and generosity have a ripple effect. When one person gives back, it can inspire others to do the same. Leading by example can create a positive cycle of compassion and altruism within a community or society.

8. Addressing Social Issues: Giving back plays a crucial role in addressing social inequalities and supporting vulnerable populations. It helps bridge gaps in access to resources and opportunities, making a significant impact on various social issues, such as poverty, education, healthcare, and environmental conservation.
9. Legacy and Long-Term Impact: The impact of giving back extends far beyond the immediate moment. Charitable contributions and community initiatives can leave a lasting legacy, creating a better world for future generations.
10. Cultivating Gratitude: Engaging in acts of giving can deepen feelings of gratitude for one's own circumstances and privileges. It reminds individuals of their own blessings and encourages appreciation for what they have.

The act of giving back is not limited to financial donations; it can also involve giving time, skills, expertise, or emotional support. From volunteering at local shelters to participating in environmental conservation efforts or supporting global humanitarian organizations, there are countless ways to give back and make a positive impact. By embracing the spirit of giving and incorporating it into our lives, we can create a more compassionate, connected, and fulfilling world for everyone.

Seven

THE FOURTH SECRET

"PURSUIT OF PASSIONS," emphasizes the importance of investing time and energy into hobbies, interests, and activities that bring joy, fulfillment, and a sense of purpose to one's life. Pursuing passions is about engaging in activities that resonate with your core values and personal preferences, leading to a more meaningful and enriched existence.

Key aspects of pursuing passions:

1. Self-Expression: Pursuing passions allows individuals to express themselves creatively and authentically. It provides an outlet for self-discovery and personal growth.
2. Joy and Fulfillment: Engaging in activities that are personally meaningful can lead to feelings of joy, fulfillment, and a sense of accomplishment.
3. Flow State: Pursuing passions often involves activities

that induce a "flow state," where individuals become fully absorbed in the task at hand, experiencing a state of optimal performance and enjoyment.

4. Stress Relief: Immersing oneself in enjoyable activities can serve as a form of stress relief, offering a break from daily challenges and worries.
5. Personal Growth: The pursuit of passions involves continuous learning and skill development, leading to personal growth and a sense of achievement.
6. Increased Motivation: Being passionate about something can boost motivation and drive to overcome obstacles and achieve goals.
7. Connection with Others: Sharing passions with like-minded individuals can foster connections and a sense of belonging to a community.
8. Improved Well-Being: Engaging in activities that bring joy and meaning can contribute to improved mental, emotional, and even physical well-being.

Tips for pursuing passions:

1. Identify Your Passions: Reflect on activities that genuinely bring you joy and make you lose track of time. These could be creative pursuits, sports, hobbies, or any other activity that sparks excitement.
2. Make Time: Prioritize and allocate time for pursuing your passions, even amid busy schedules. It can be as simple as setting aside a few minutes each day or dedicating specific days for your hobbies.
3. Overcome Barriers: Address any barriers that prevent you from pursuing your passions, such as self-doubt, fear of

failure, or time constraints.

4. Experiment and Explore: Don't be afraid to try new activities and explore different interests. Passion may emerge from unexpected places.

5. Embrace Learning: Embrace the learning process and view challenges as opportunities to grow and improve in your chosen pursuits.

6. Balance and Moderation: While pursuing passions is essential, maintaining a balance with other aspects of life is equally crucial. Find ways to integrate your passions into your daily routine without neglecting other responsibilities.

By pursuing passions, individuals can infuse their lives with purpose, joy, and a sense of fulfillment. It adds depth to daily experiences and contributes to a more vibrant and rewarding life journey. Remember, it's never too late to discover new passions or reignite old ones, as life's journey is an ongoing exploration of what brings meaning and happiness.

Of course! The pursuit of passions is a deeply personal and trans formative journey that allows individuals to connect with their authentic selves and cultivate a fulfilling and purposeful life. Let's delve further into the significance and benefits of pursuing passions, along with additional tips for integrating them into daily life.

The Importance of Pursuing Passions:

1. Self-Discovery and Authenticity: Engaging in activities that resonate with your passions can lead to a deeper understanding of yourself and your unique interests. By embracing your passions, you foster a greater sense of

authenticity and align your actions with your true self.

2. A Source of Joy and Fulfillment: Pursuing passions brings a sense of joy and fulfillment that can be difficult to find elsewhere. When you do what you love, you infuse enthusiasm into your everyday experiences, making life more vibrant and enjoyable.

3. Increased Motivation and Resilience: Passion fuels motivation, enabling you to persevere through challenges and setbacks. The drive to improve in your chosen pursuits pushes you to overcome obstacles, fostering resilience and a growth mindset.

4. Stress Reduction and Well-Being: Engaging in activities that bring joy can act as a form of stress relief, promoting emotional well-being and mental relaxation.

5. Creativity and Innovation: Passionate individuals often approach their hobbies and interests with creativity and innovation. Exploring new ideas and pushing boundaries can lead to personal breakthroughs and unique perspectives.

6. Enhanced Focus and Flow State: Pursuing passions often leads to a state of "flow" - a mental state of complete absorption in an activity where time seems to fly by. This heightened focus enhances productivity and performance.

7. Meaning and Purpose: The pursuit of passions adds depth and meaning to life. It provides a sense of purpose and direction, giving you something to look forward to and invest your time and energy in.

Tips for Embracing Passion:

1. Reflect and Explore: Take time to reflect on your interests,

childhood hobbies, and activities that excite you. Explore new experiences to discover potential passions.

2. Overcome Self-Doubt: Recognize and challenge any self-doubt or limiting beliefs that might hold you back from embracing your passions fully.

3. Set Clear Goals: Establish clear goals related to your passions. Having specific objectives can help you stay motivated and measure your progress.

4. Create a Supportive Environment: Surround yourself with like-minded individuals who share your interests or can encourage and inspire your pursuit of passions.

5. Embrace Failure and Learning: Embrace failure as an essential part of the learning process. Understand that setbacks are opportunities to grow and improve.

6. Incorporate Passion into Your Routine: Integrate your passions into your daily life by setting aside dedicated time for them. Even small moments of engagement can make a significant impact over time.

7. Embrace Balance: While passion is vital, finding balance with other aspects of life is essential. Prioritize your passions without neglecting other responsibilities.

8. Share Your Passion: Share your passion with others, whether through teaching, volunteering, or collaborating on projects. It creates opportunities for connection and inspiration.

Remember, passions can evolve over time, and it's natural to explore various interests at different stages of life. Embrace the journey of discovering and nurturing your passions, as it leads to a more authentic, joyful, and meaningful existence. By integrating your passions into your life, you embark on a path of self-discovery and personal growth that enriches both your well-being and the lives of those around you.

Eight

THE FIFTH SECRET

"EMBRACING CHANGE," underscores the importance of accepting and adapting to the constant evolution and unpredictability of life. It involves developing a flexible and resilient mindset to navigate through transitions, challenges, and new experiences with a positive and open outlook.

Key aspects of embracing change:

1. Adaptability: Embracing change requires the ability to adjust and adapt to new circumstances, whether they are related to personal life, work, relationships, or external factors.

2. Growth and Learning: Change often brings opportunities for growth and learning. Embracing change as a chance for personal development can lead to new skills, insights, and perspectives.

3. Letting Go of the Past: Accepting change involves letting go of attachments to the past and embracing the idea that life is constantly evolving.
4. Optimism and Resilience: A positive outlook and resilience are essential for coping with change and bouncing back from adversity.
5. Flexibility and Openness: Being open-minded and flexible allows you to embrace new possibilities and approaches that arise from change.
6. Finding Opportunities: Change can create opportunities for new experiences, relationships, and paths that may not have been apparent before.
7. Embracing Uncertainty: Recognizing that change brings uncertainty can lead to a mindset of curiosity and exploration rather than fear.
8. Self-Reflection: Embracing change encourages self-reflection, helping you understand your values, goals, and aspirations as they evolve over time.

Benefits of embracing change:

1. Personal Growth: Change often requires stepping out of comfort zones, which can lead to personal growth, self-discovery, and increased self-confidence.
2. Enhanced Problem-Solving Skills: Adapting to change fosters problem-solving skills, as you navigate new situations and challenges.
3. Expanded Resilience: Embracing change builds resilience, enabling you to better cope with life's ups and downs.
4. Improved Emotional Intelligence: Navigating change involves understanding and managing emotions effectively,

leading to improved emotional intelligence.

5. Increased Creativity: Change can spark creativity, as you explore new possibilities and solutions.
6. Embracing Opportunities: Accepting change opens doors to new opportunities and experiences that may have remained hidden in a static and rigid mindset.
7. Strengthened Relationships: The ability to adapt to change can strengthen relationships by fostering empathy and understanding.

Tips for Embracing Change:

1. Mindfulness: Practicing mindfulness can help you stay present and grounded during times of change, reducing anxiety about the future.
2. Self-Compassion: Be kind to yourself during periods of change, understanding that it's natural to experience a mix of emotions.
3. Focus on What You Can Control: Concentrate on aspects of change you can influence, and accept the aspects you cannot.
4. Seek Support: Talk to friends, family, or seek professional support if you find change overwhelming.
5. Embrace Learning: View change as an opportunity to learn and grow, even if it comes with challenges.
6. Stay Open to New Perspectives: Embrace change with an open mind and willingness to consider new perspectives.

Embracing change is an ongoing process that requires self-awareness, flexibility, and a positive mindset. By cultivating the ability to adapt to life's changes, you equip yourself to face the unknown with courage and resilience, fostering personal growth and a more enriched and fulfilling life journey.

Certainly! Here are additional insights and benefits related to embracing change:

1. Increased Confidence: Successfully navigating through change and adapting to new situations can boost self-confidence and self-efficacy.
2. Empowerment: Embracing change empowers individuals to take control of their lives and make proactive decisions about their future.
3. Embracing Diversity: Change often brings diversity into our lives, exposing us to different perspectives, cultures, and ideas, fostering tolerance and understanding.
4. Innovation and Creativity: Embracing change can stimulate innovation and creativity as individuals explore new approaches and solutions.
5. Finding Hidden Strengths: Facing change can reveal hidden strengths and abilities that may not have been apparent during times of stability.
6. Overcoming Fear: Embracing change can help individuals confront and overcome their fears, leading to personal growth and increased resilience.
7. Building Coping Strategies: Successfully adapting to change builds a repertoire of coping strategies, making individuals better equipped to handle future challenges.
8. Embracing Life Transitions: Life is full of transitions, such as moving to a new city, changing jobs, or starting a family. Embracing change prepares individuals for these significant life transitions.
9. Growth Mindset: Embracing change aligns with a growth

mindset, the belief that challenges and failures are opportunities for growth and learning.

10. Developing Emotional Agility: The ability to navigate changing emotions during times of change fosters emotional agility and emotional intelligence.

Tips for Embracing Change:

1. Cultivate Self-Awareness: Understand your reactions to change and how it impacts your emotions and behavior.
2. Practice Mindfulness and Acceptance: Accept the reality of change and practice mindfulness to stay grounded in the present moment.
3. Create a Supportive Environment: Surround yourself with a supportive network of friends, family, or colleagues who can provide encouragement and understanding.
4. Embrace Change Incrementally: Embracing small changes can build confidence and prepare you for more significant transformations.
5. View Change as an Opportunity: Shift your perspective to see change as an opportunity for growth and positive transformation.
6. Learn from Previous Experiences: Reflect on past changes you have experienced and identify the valuable lessons learned.
7. Take Proactive Steps: Rather than resisting change, take proactive steps to adapt and find constructive solutions.
8. Set Realistic Expectations: Understand that change takes time, and it is normal to face challenges along the way.

Embracing change is an ongoing journey that requires continuous effort and self-awareness. By recognizing change as an integral part of life and embracing it with openness and courage, individuals can tap into their inner resilience and personal growth potential. Ultimately, the ability to embrace change allows us to navigate life's uncertainties with grace and confidence, leading to a more fulfilled and meaningful existence.

Certainly! Let's explore some additional aspects and considerations related to embracing change:

1. Learning from Failure: Embracing change involves recognizing that failure is a natural part of the process. Rather than fearing failure, view it as an opportunity for growth and learning.
2. Flexibility in Planning: Embracing change requires flexibility in planning and a willingness to adjust goals and strategies as circumstances evolve.
3. Cultivating Patience: Change may not happen overnight, and the process can be gradual. Cultivating patience allows individuals to navigate change with a steady and calm approach.
4. Balancing Stability and Change: Embracing change does not mean completely abandoning stability and routine. It's about finding a balance between adaptability and maintaining aspects of life that bring comfort and structure.
5. Embracing Career Changes: Career transitions can be significant life changes. Embrace opportunities for career growth, reevaluation of professional goals, and exploring new paths.
6. Self-Reflection and Self-Care: During times of change, take moments for self-reflection and self-care to better

understand your emotions and needs.

7. Embracing Aging and Life Stages: As life progresses, embracing changes associated with aging and different life stages can lead to acceptance and a positive outlook on the journey.
8. Resisting Complacency: Embracing change prevents falling into complacency or stagnation. It encourages continuous growth and development.
9. Embracing Cultural and Technological Changes: Societal changes, such as advancements in technology and cultural shifts, require openness to adapt and evolve.
10. Mentorship and Support: Seek mentorship or guidance from individuals who have experienced similar changes. Surround yourself with a supportive community to navigate transitions.
11. Celebrating Progress: Acknowledge and celebrate milestones achieved during periods of change, no matter how small they may seem.
12. Fostering a Growth Mindset: Adopt a growth mindset that views challenges and setbacks as opportunities for learning and improvement.

Remember that change is a constant part of life, and embracing it is a journey that unfolds uniquely for each person. By embracing change with a positive attitude, openness, and a willingness to learn, individuals can develop resilience, courage, and adaptability, leading to a more fulfilling and purposeful life. Embracing change as an integral part of the human experience can be a trans formative and empowering process, enabling individuals to embrace the beauty of life's uncertainties and navigate the future with confidence and optimism.

Nine

MEANING OF SECRET

The term "secret" typically refers to information, knowledge, or something kept hidden or undisclosed from others. It can be a piece of information that is not widely known or intentionally kept private, shared only with a select few or kept confidential for various reasons.

In the context of the conversation, the word "secret" was used metaphorically to describe five interesting and insightful aspects related to living a good life. These aspects were referred to as "secrets" to emphasize their significance and the potential impact they can have on enhancing well-being and happiness.

In a broader sense, "secret" can also be associated with mystery, confidentiality, and exclusivity. However, when used in a positive context, it often refers to valuable information or insights that can bring about positive changes in one's life or the lives of others.

Certainly! In a broader context, "secret" can have various

meanings and implications. Here are some additional perspectives on the term:

1. Confidentiality and Privacy: A secret can refer to confidential or private information shared between individuals or within a group, with the understanding that it should not be disclosed to others without permission.
2. Hidden Knowledge: Secrets can involve knowledge or information that is deliberately concealed, whether for personal, professional, or strategic reasons.
3. Intrigue and Mystery: The notion of a secret can evoke a sense of mystery and intrigue, as it implies something undisclosed or not fully understood.
4. Symbolism: Secrets can be symbolic, representing underlying truths, emotions, or motivations that are not readily apparent on the surface.
5. Power and Control: In certain contexts, secrets can be used as a tool to maintain power or control over others, as the withholding of information can influence decisions and behavior.
6. Surprise and Delight: Secrets can also be associated with pleasant surprises or hidden gifts, adding an element of excitement and delight to certain situations.
7. Uncovering Truth: In storytelling, secrets often play a pivotal role in driving the narrative forward, as characters strive to uncover hidden truths or solve mysteries.
8. Personal Insights: On a personal level, individuals may use the term "secret" to describe unique or deeply held insights about themselves or their life experiences.

It's important to recognize that not all secrets are positive or constructive. Some secrets may cause harm or perpetuate dishonesty, leading to negative consequences in personal relationships or broader contexts. Open communication, trust, and ethical considerations play crucial roles in how secrets are perceived and managed.

Ultimately, the concept of a secret can evoke a wide range of emotions and reactions, and its interpretation may vary based on cultural, societal, and individual perspectives. In a positive light, secrets can hold the potential for intrigue, surprise, and personal growth, while in a negative context, they can lead to mistrust and disharmony.

Ten

Summary

1. Gratitude: Cultivating a practice of gratitude involves being thankful and appreciative for the positive aspects of life, leading to a more positive outlook and emotional well-being.
2. Mindfulness: Practicing mindfulness means being fully present in the moment, without judgment, which can reduce stress and enhance self-awareness, leading to a more fulfilling and balanced life.
3. Giving Back: Engaging in acts of kindness and giving back to others fosters a sense of purpose and fulfillment, creating a positive impact on both the giver and the recipient.
4. Pursuit of Passions: Investing time in hobbies and interests that bring joy and fulfillment allows for self-expression, personal growth, and a greater sense of purpose in life.

5. Embracing Change: Embracing change involves accepting and adapting to life's uncertainties and challenges, leading to personal growth, resilience, and an optimistic outlook on life.

By incorporating these five secrets into one's life, individuals can enhance their well-being, find meaning, and create a more fulfilling and balanced existence, contributing to a GOOD LIFE.

Eleven

Conclusion

In conclusion, the pursuit of a GOOD LIFE involves embracing essential aspects that contribute to overall well-being, fulfillment, and happiness. The five secrets—gratitude, mindfulness, giving back, pursuit of passions, and embracing change—serve as guiding principles to achieve a more meaningful and balanced life.

Gratitude fosters positivist and appreciation for life's blessings, while mindfulness enables individuals to stay present and attuned to their experiences. Giving back creates a sense of purpose and interconnections with others, and pursuing passions allows for self-expression and personal growth.

Finally, embracing change with an open mind and resilience enables individuals to navigate life's uncertainties and challenges with grace, leading to personal growth and a positive outlook on the future.

By integrating these secrets into daily life, individuals can enhance their overall well-being, cultivate stronger relationships, and lead a more fulfilling and purposeful life. Remember, the journey towards a GOOD LIFE is unique to each individual, and by actively incorporating these principles, one can create a life of meaning, joy, and contentment

Twelve

Chapter 12

www.ingramcontent.com/pod-product-compliance
Lightning Source LLC
Chambersburg PA
CBHW060857260726
48661CB00008B/3317